How To Shape A Perfect Smile

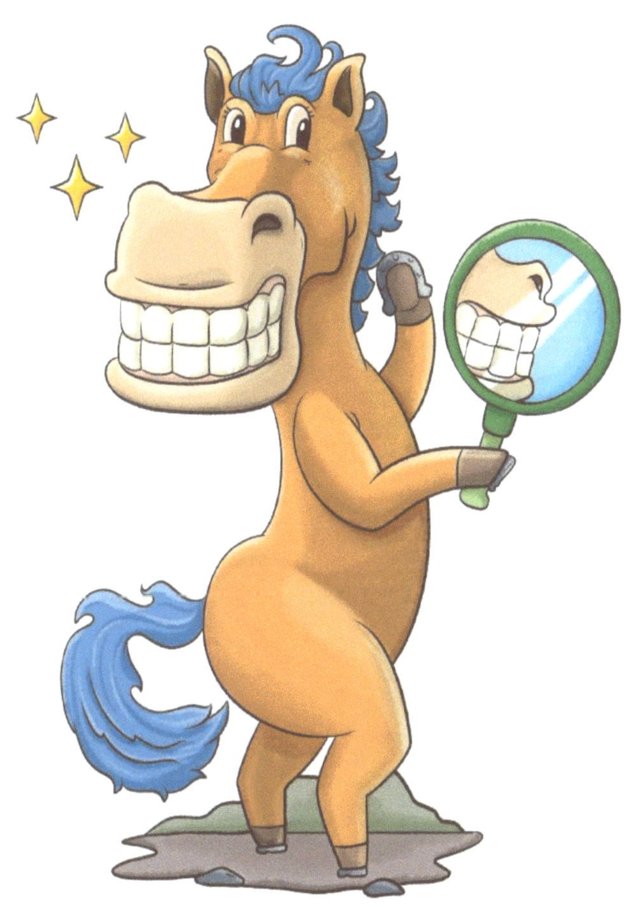

Nibras Sharif, DDS

Illustrated By Dom Sadehawa

Dear parents,

I love seeing people smile from their hearts and to me all smiles are beautiful. However, healthy habits help a child develop healthy teeth and a healthy body. Ever since I changed the smile of my daughter by helping her recognize her habits, I have wanted all children to know the importance of their mouth habits.

This book is written to help recognize common unhealthy mouth habits in children aged between 4-11 years. This book will help your child understand how moving the mouth while breathing or eating is important for the growth of their face. If you recognize any of these habits in your child, discuss it with them. If you notice a persistent habit that is changing your child's teeth or face, please address them with your dental health team as soon as you can.

Dedicated to all the children of the world. May you never stop smiling!

There are many ways you can change your smile
And even the shape of your face

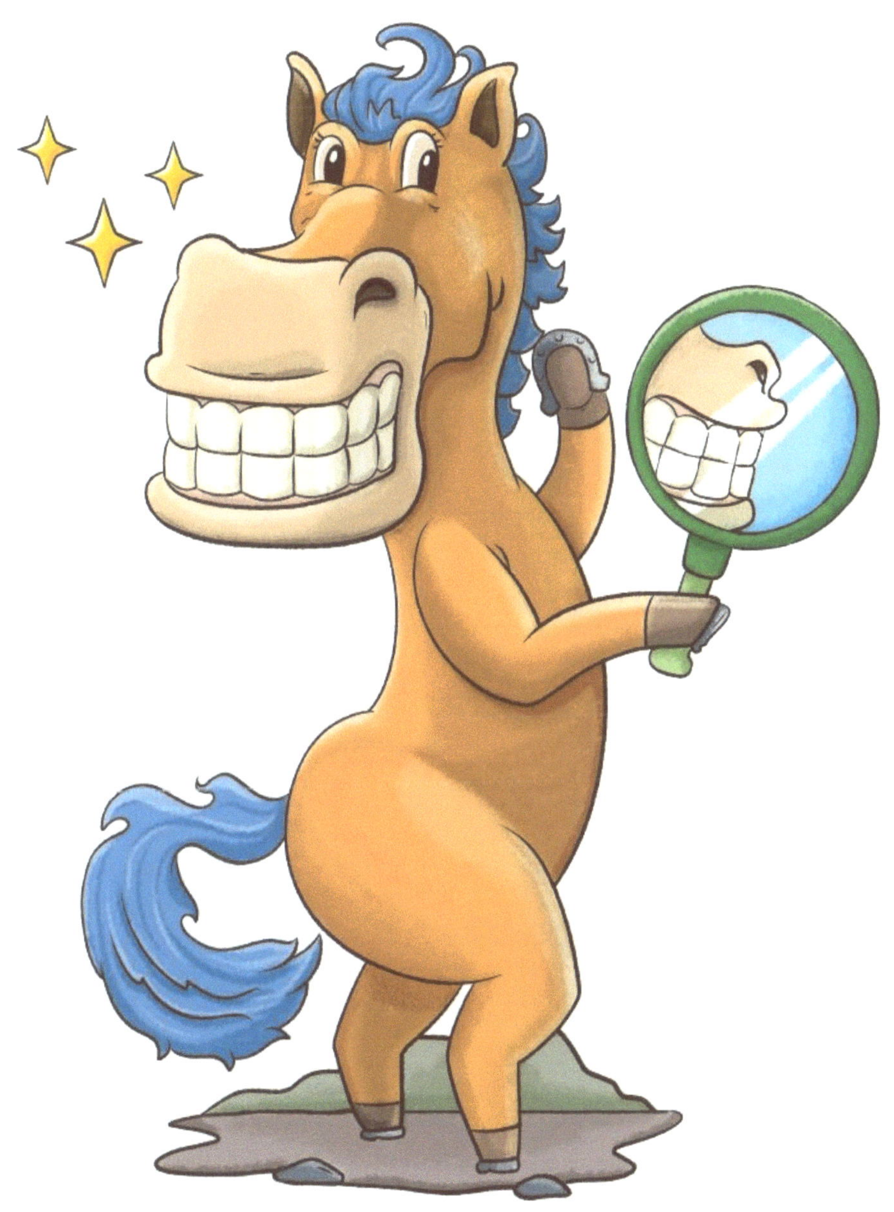

The way your face grows can be changed by how you use your teeth, muscles, and bones.

If you always pant and breathe from your mouth,
You will drop your tongue way down low
Your face will look long
And your breath will feel short

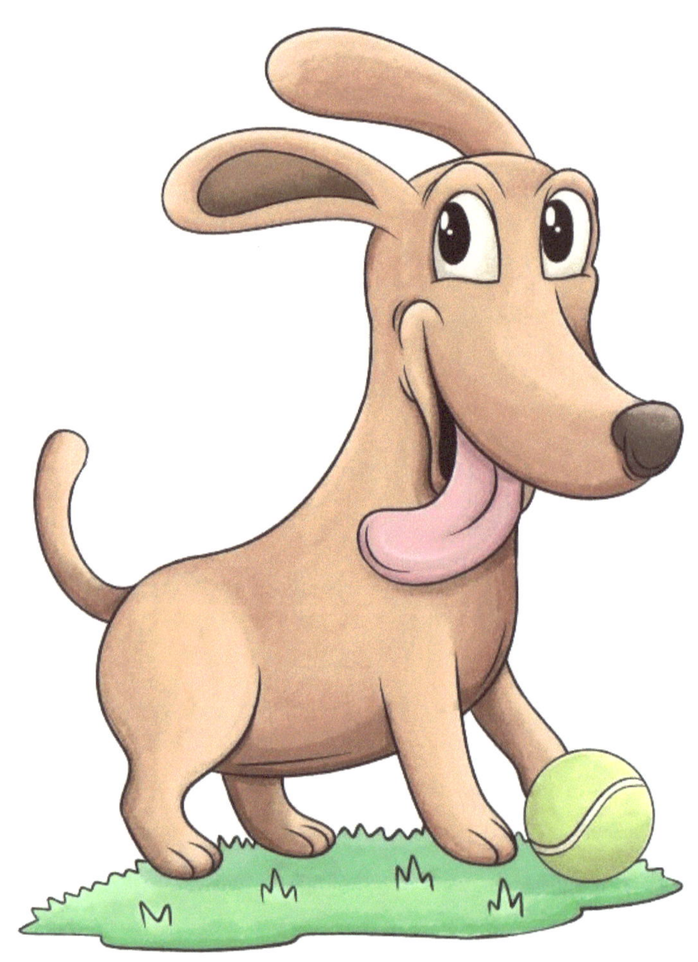

Dogs pant when they are feeling hot or need more air. This causes their tongues to stick out and their jaws to be pushed down. In humans, mouth breathing will also cause the tongue to fall low and face to grow long. Mouth breathing also makes our breath shallow and fast. We usually feel more tired and tense when we breathe from our mouths.

If you forget to use your nose,
It may shrivel and shrink
Your bite may look upside down
Like a Piranha fish with a frown

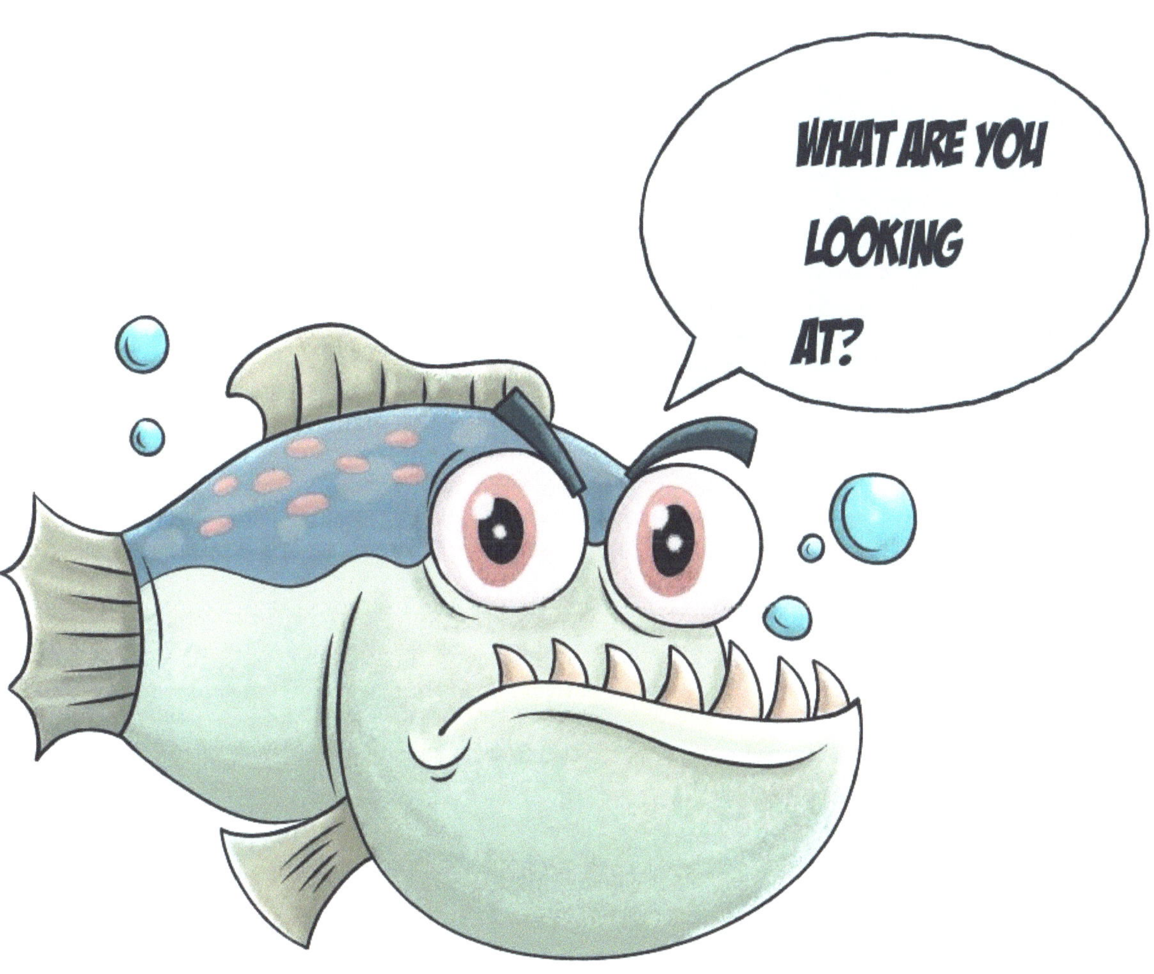

Breathing from the mouth all the time can make your nose and top jaw stay small while your bottom jaw grows big and strong. Your face may look just like a Piranha fish.

Then you will snore so high
That your ears will twitch at night

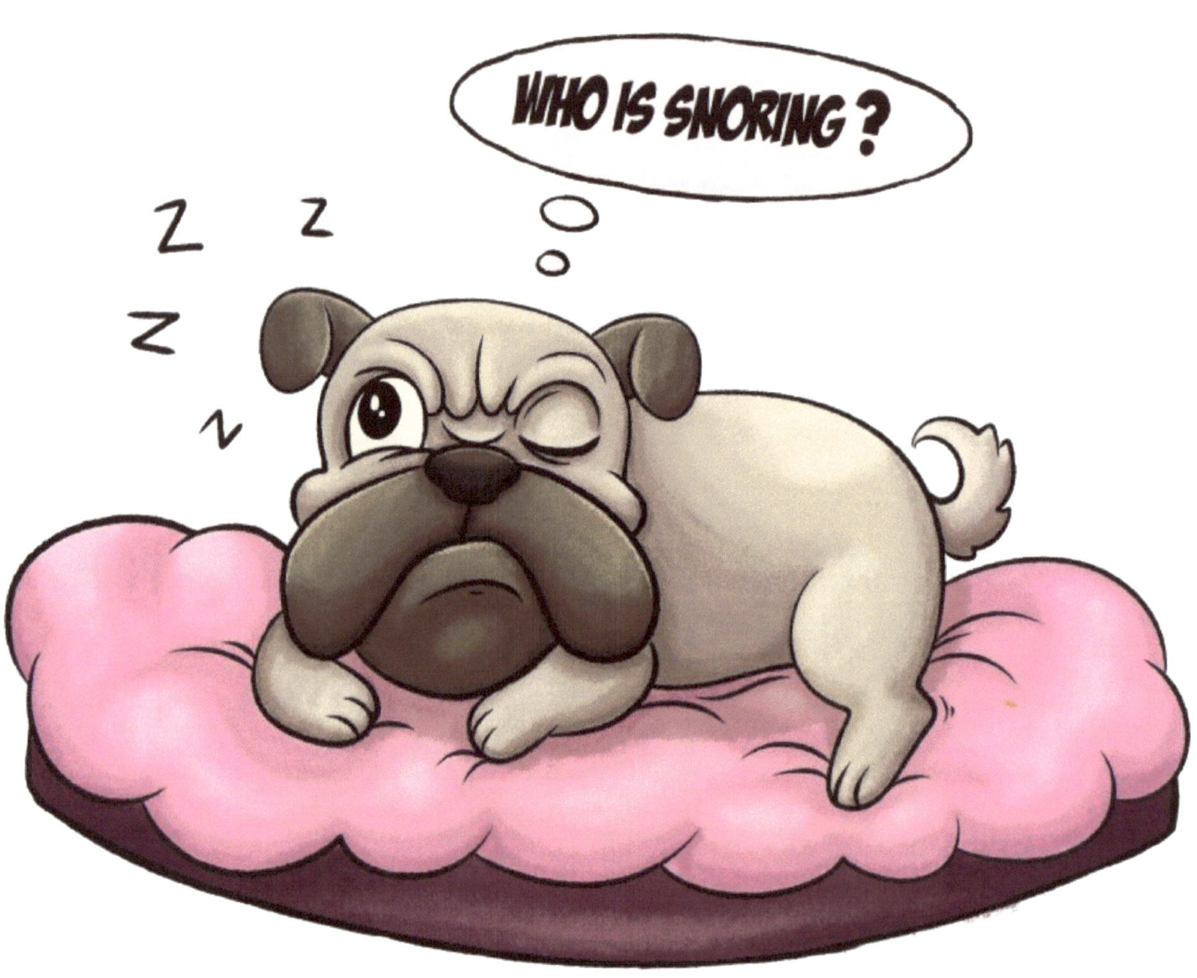

Pugs snore loudly because they breathe through their mouths and have large bottom jaws. If you breathe through your mouth, you will also make loud snoring sounds.

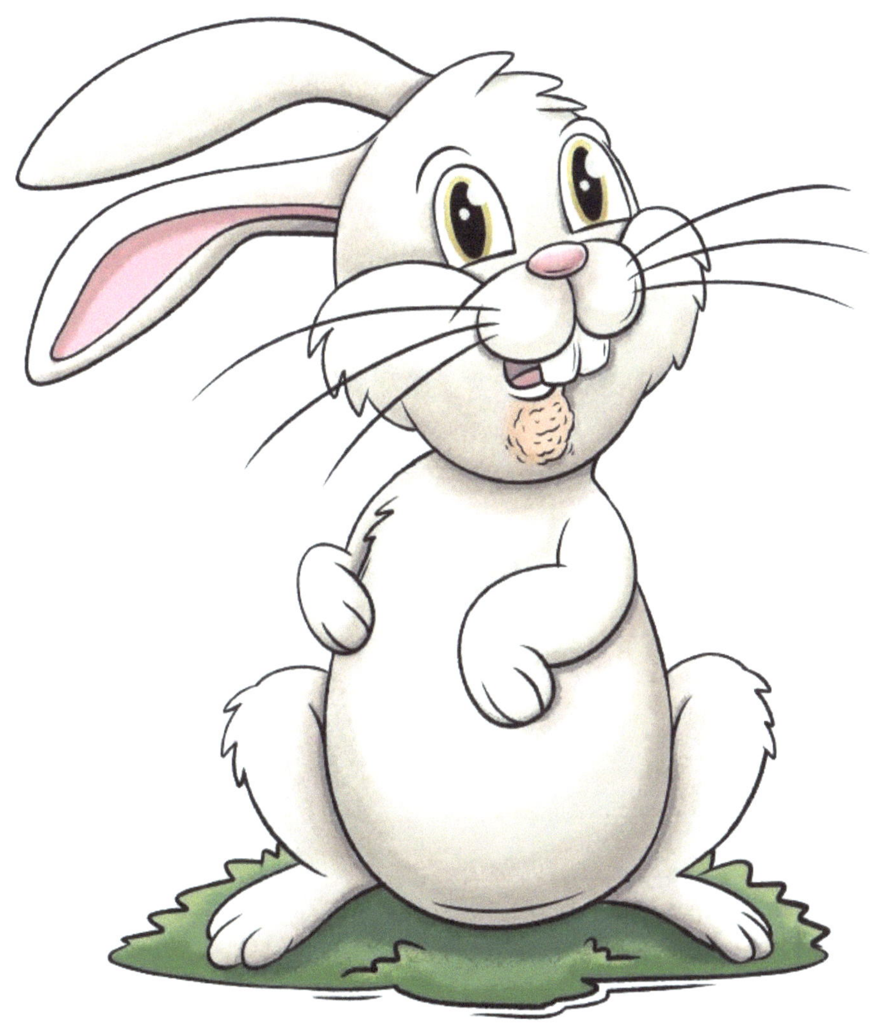

If you eat with a wrinkle on your lips,
You will grow a bunny chin with orange peel skin

The chin and teeth of a rabbit look different because rabbits use their lips to push food back into their mouths. If you use your lips to eat and swallow, the chin muscles will start to look wrinkled and puckered like orange peel.

If every time you gulp down,
Your tongue peeks out like a clown
Your teeth will grow apart
Until you can't chew or bite

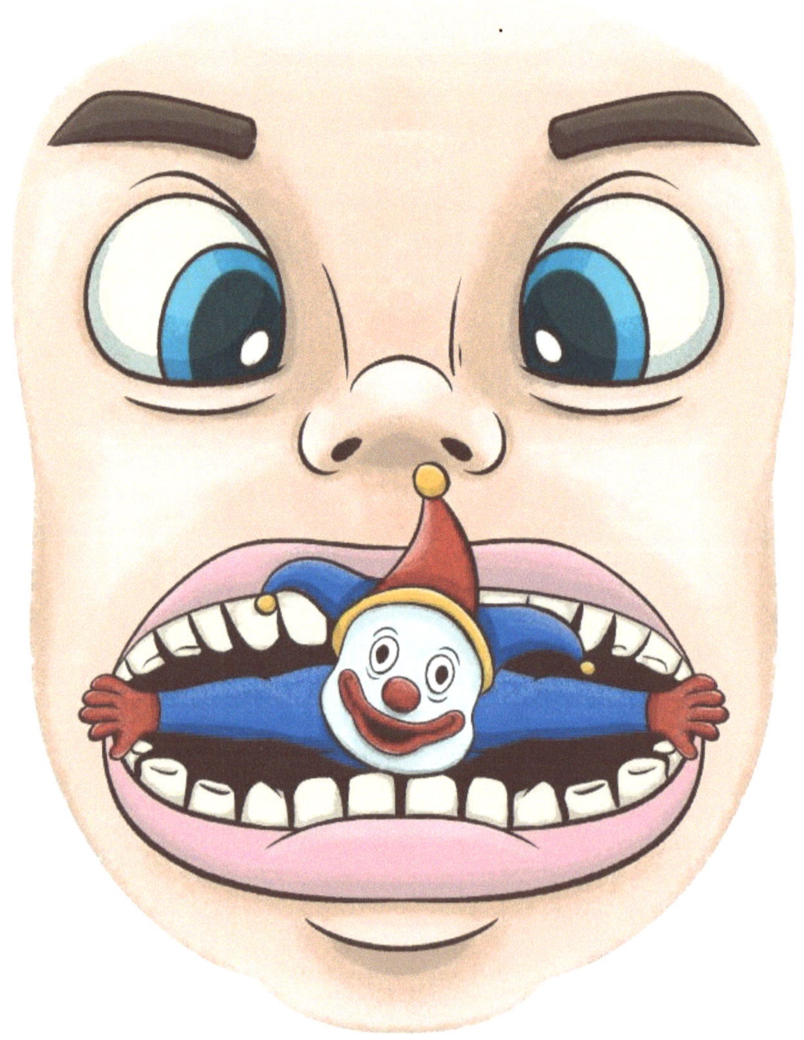

When swallowing, the tongue tip should move up and touch the roof of
the mouth only (the hard, top part of your mouth). The tongue should
never touch your front or side teeth or it will push them out.

If you keep sucking your lips,
You will push out your front teeth
Until you have a beaver face

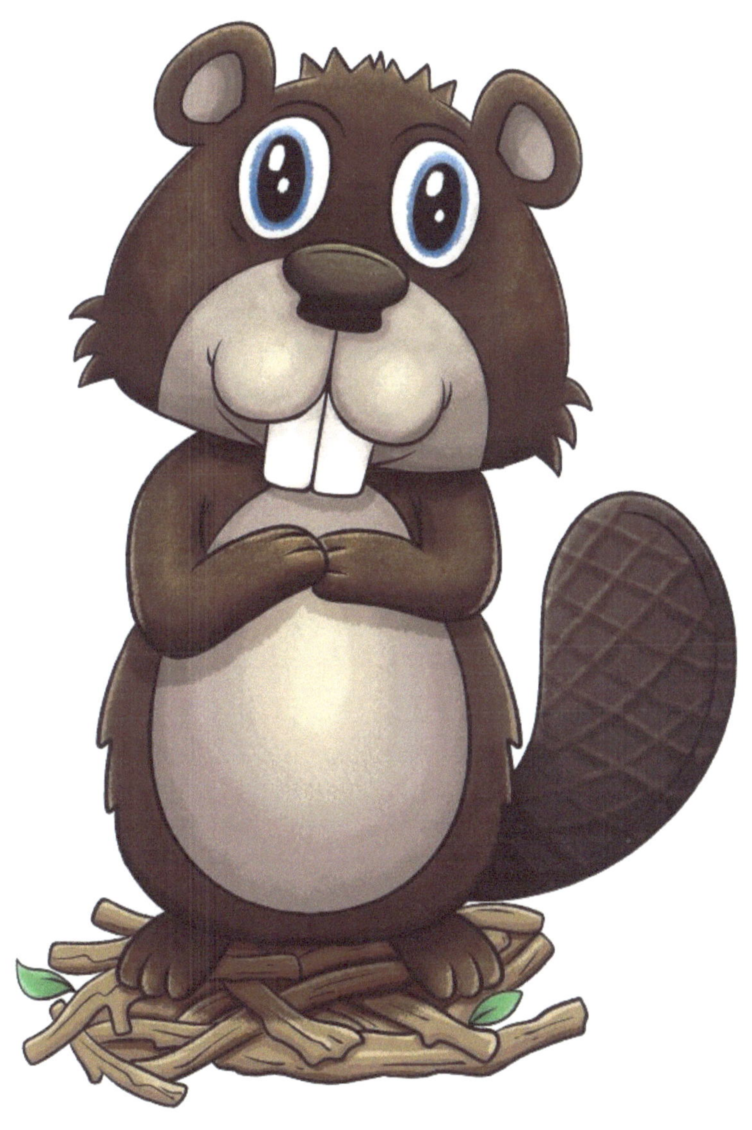

Beavers are famous for their large flat buck teeth. The beaver sucks
its lower lips so it can chew underwater. If you suck your lips, you will
also push your front teeth.

Don't bite or lick your lips
They will grow sore and big
Like an Orangutan wearing lipstick

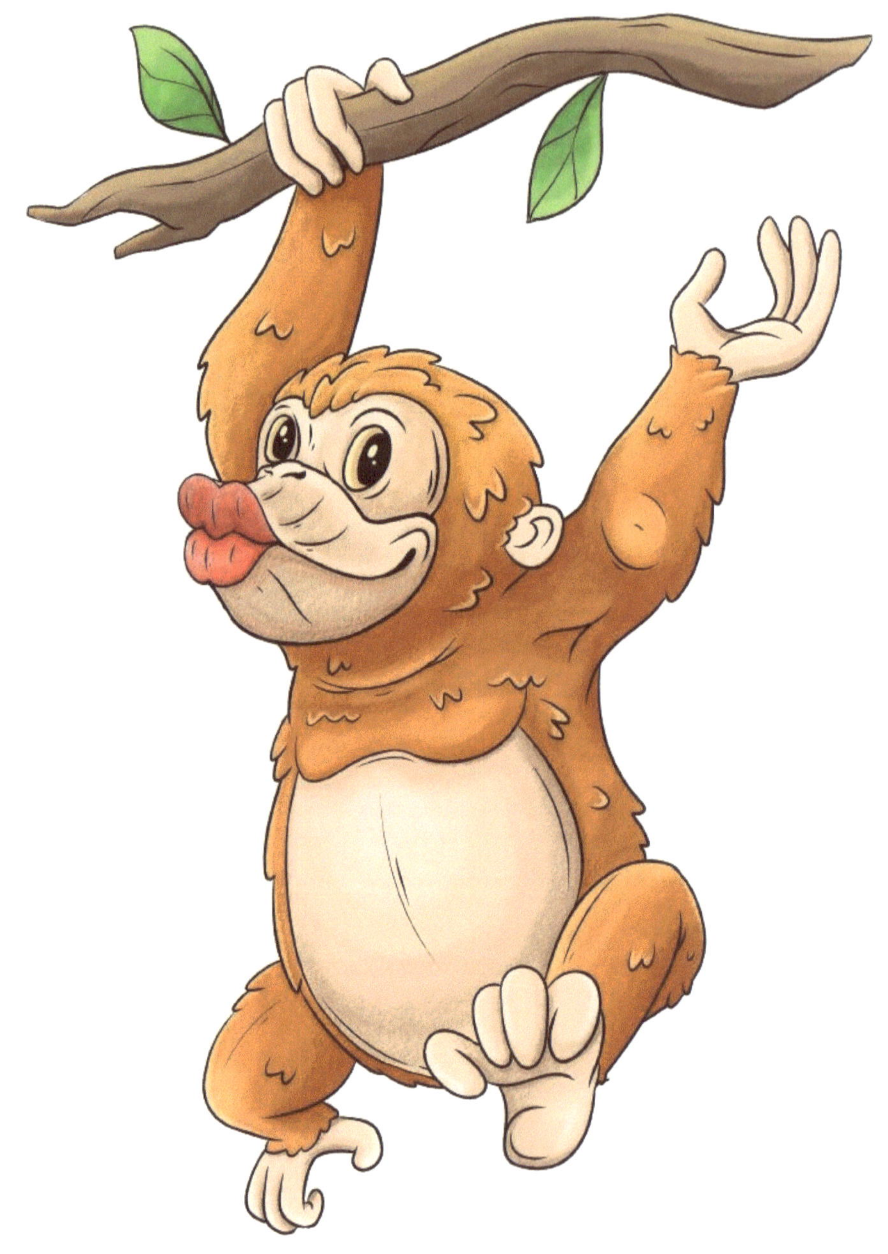

Orangutans use their lips to show their emotions. Humans also bite their lips when they are nervous, tired, or have dry lips especially in the winter. This habit can cause damage to your lips and teeth.

If you like to Chew on things,
Pencils, fingers, or your thumb
Your teeth will break and spread apart
Looking jumbled up with gaps

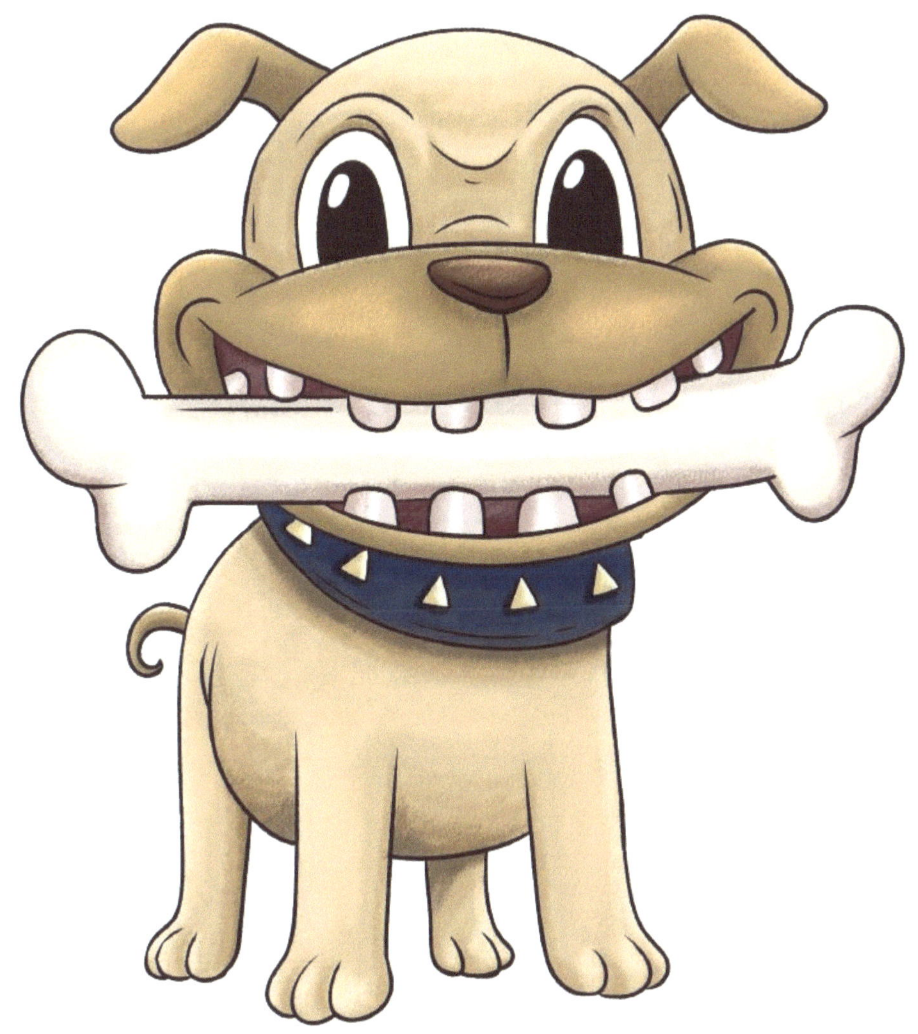

Puppies and human babies start to chew on things when they get
teeth. However, chewing habits on things other than food can change
the shape of your teeth and push them apart.

If you like to grind your teeth,
When you are bored or thinking deep
Bit by bit they will fade and break
Until all you have is stumps and big gums

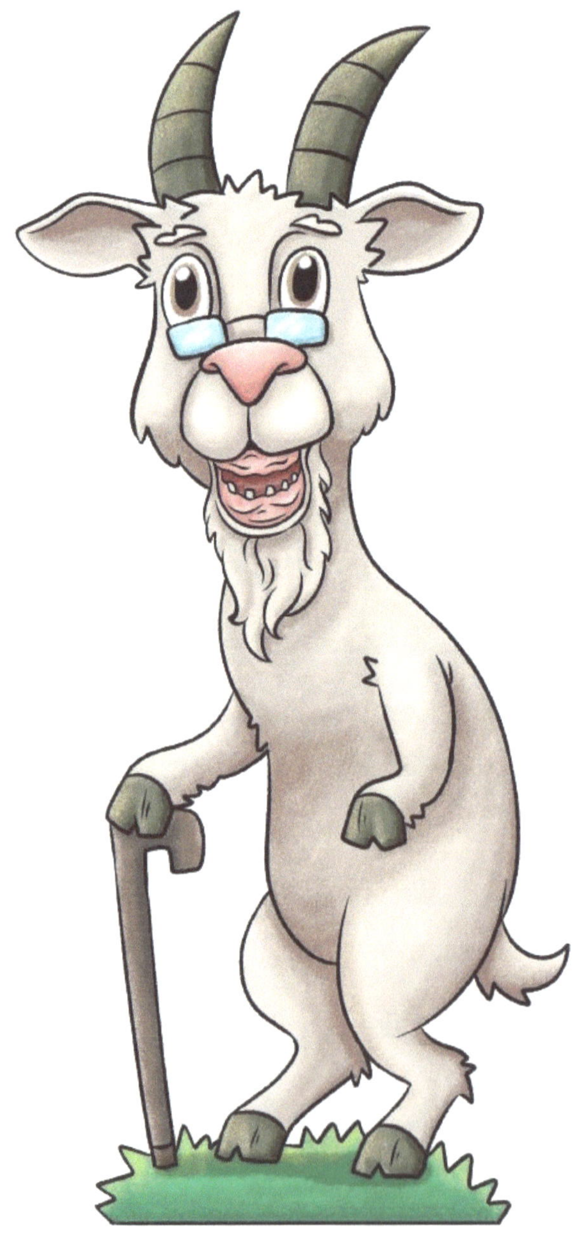

Goats grind their teeth when they are bored or sick. This can cause them to break and lose their teeth by the age of 15. Humans need their teeth to last a lifetime and maybe even more than 100 years!

My favourite are the horse's teeth
They are straight and so neat
Horses know how to swallow and bite
They breathe from their nose
And smile with delight

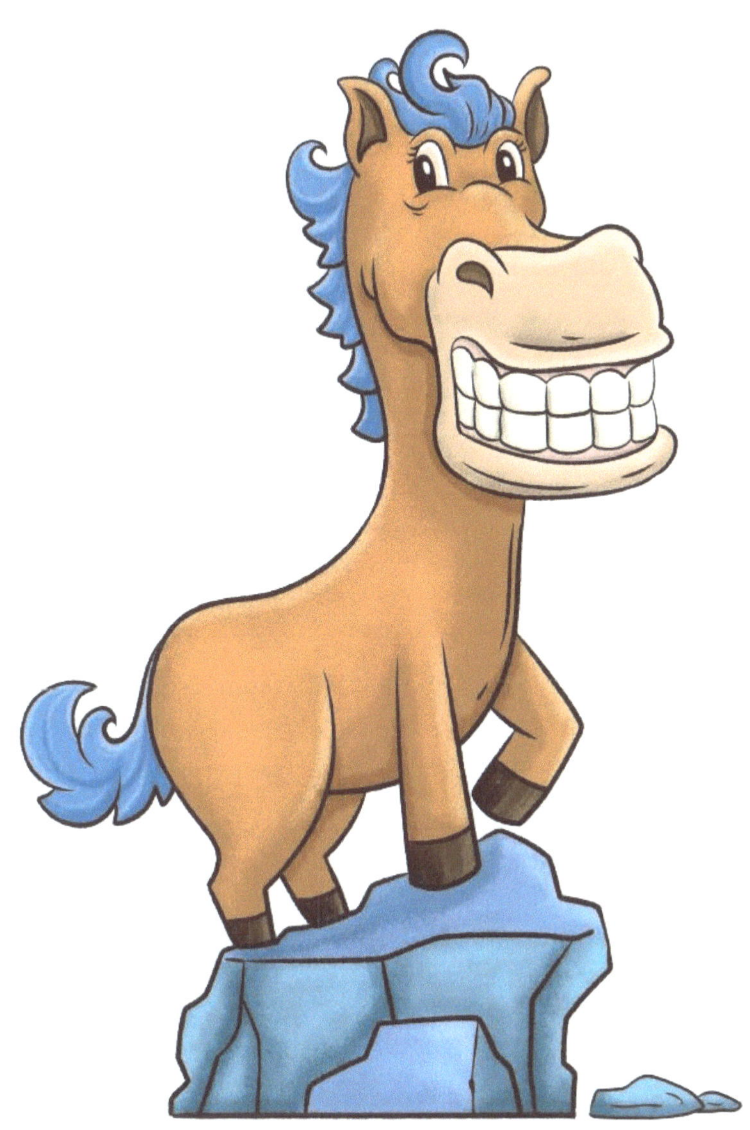

Horses are fast and elegant animals. Unlike humans, horses can only breathe from their nose and can never breathe from their mouths. Breathing through the nose gives us more energy.

If you want beautiful teeth,
And to feel at ease,
Remember to use your nose to breathe

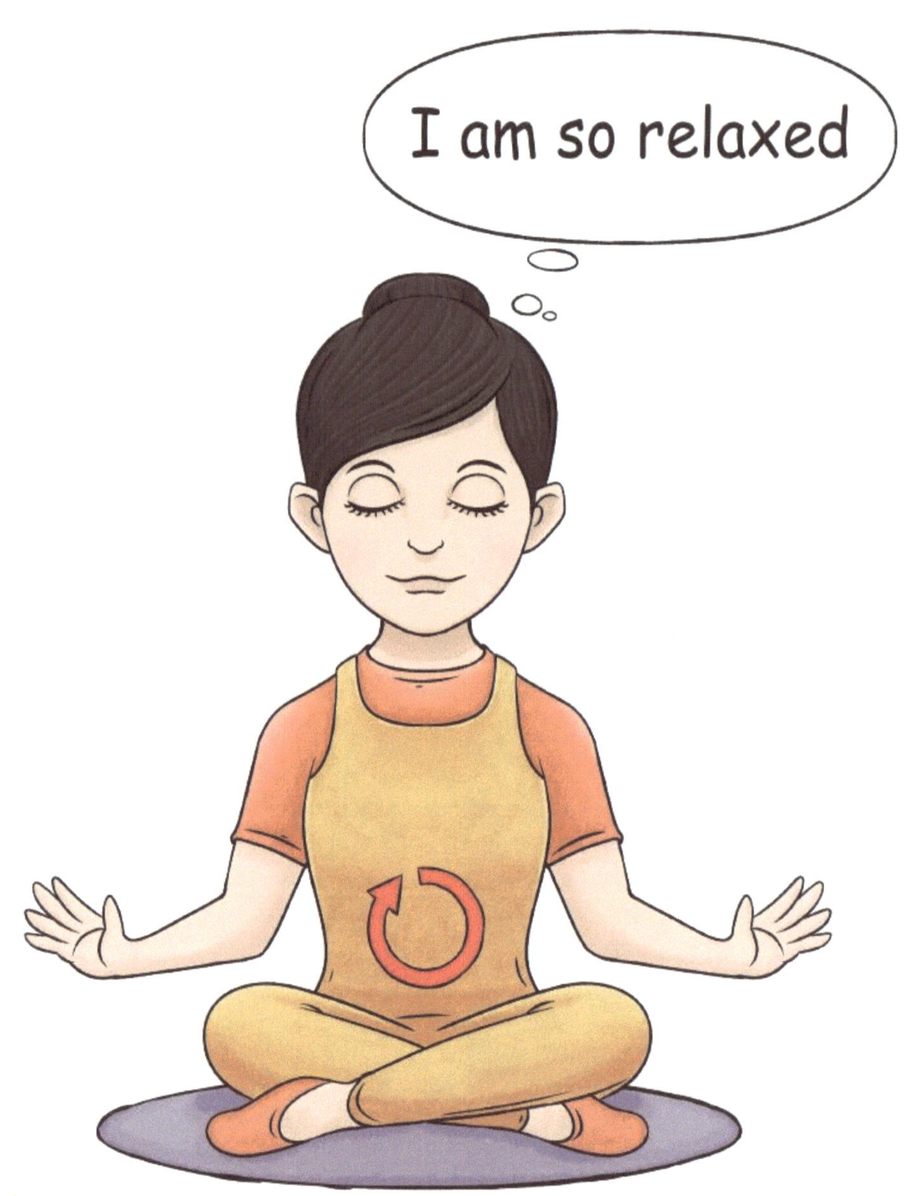

Breathing through the nose makes us feel calm and happy. The nose also cleans the air and keeps it warm for our bodies. Breathing through the mouth makes our mouth dry and can cause more cavities.

Your tongue should rest in the roof of your mouth
Snuggled up tightly in its comfy bed
So it lets you breathe and sleep in peace

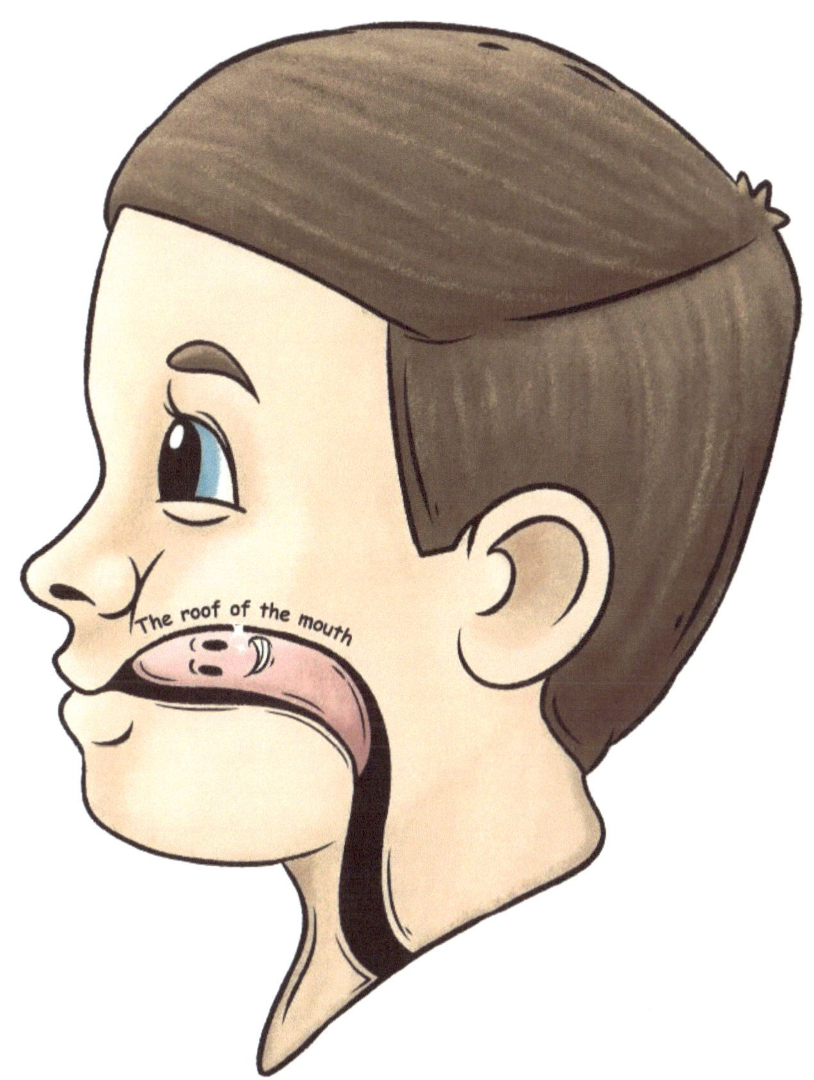

The tongue should always be touching the roof (top part) of the mouth when at rest. This position will allow your body to relax and you can also sleep better at night without snoring.

Crush your food with your back teeth
The more you chew, the better it is for you

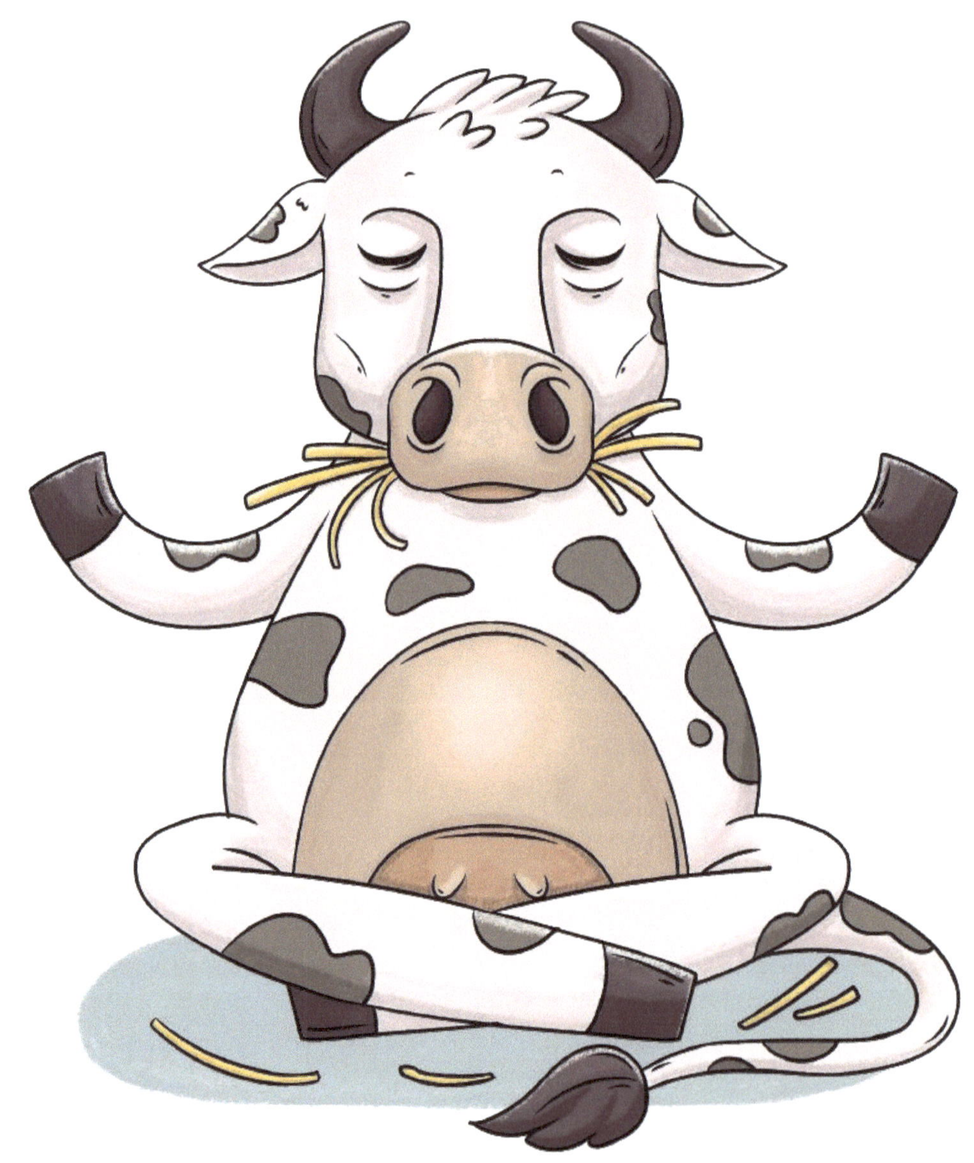

Cows chew their food twice (they chew it, swallow it, digest it, and then push it up to the mouth again for a second chew). They do this to get the maximum nutrients from food. Also, the more we learn to chew, the more nutrients (vitamins, minerals, and energy) we get out out of our food.

Move your jaws side to side
Balance your bite from left to right
Like a hippo and rhino on a sea-saw ride

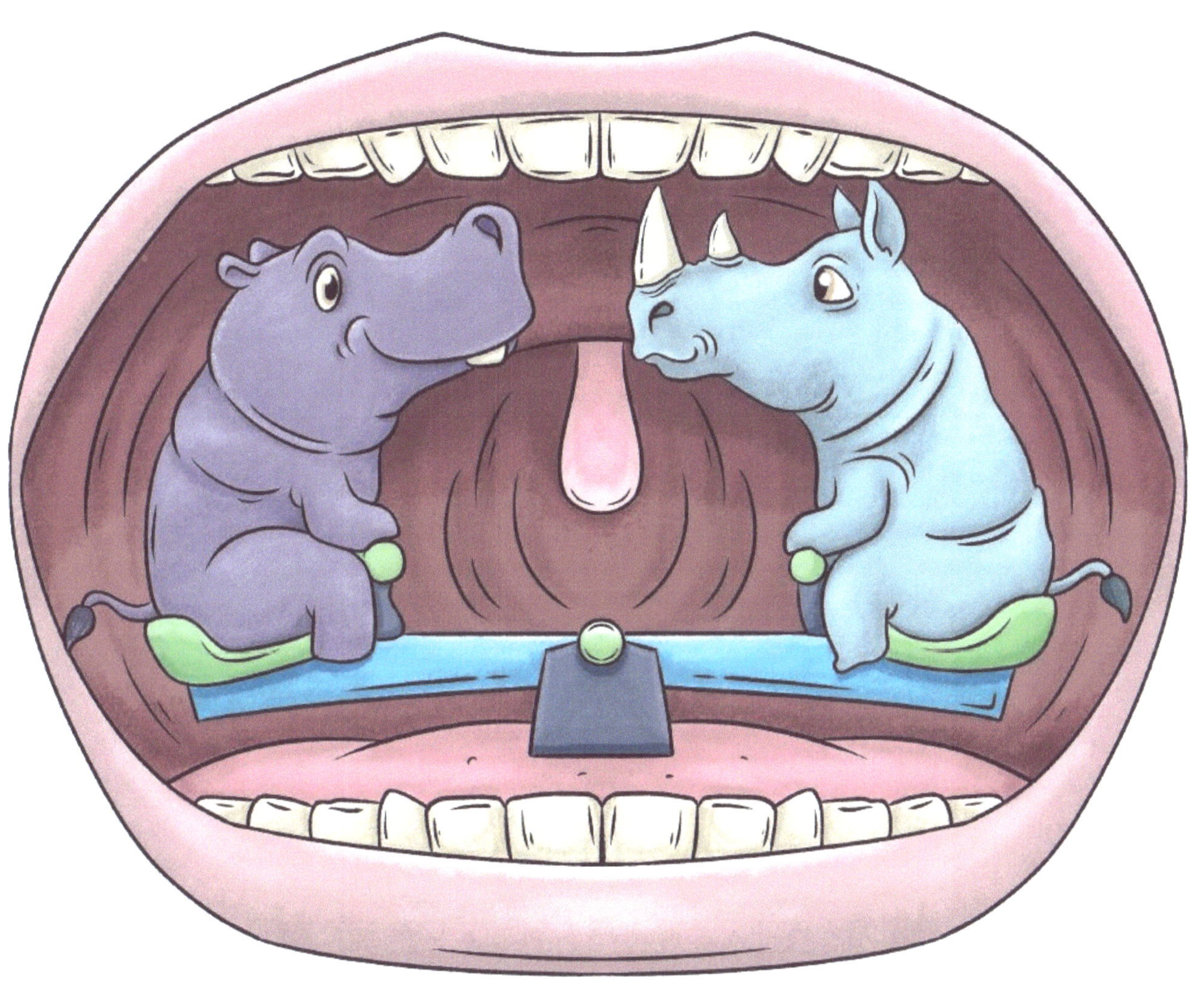

It is important to chew on both sides of the mouth and not prefer one side. Chewing on one side may cause our faces to grow crooked and tilted to our preferred chewing side.

Swallow with the muscles near your neck
Never move your lips or cheeks

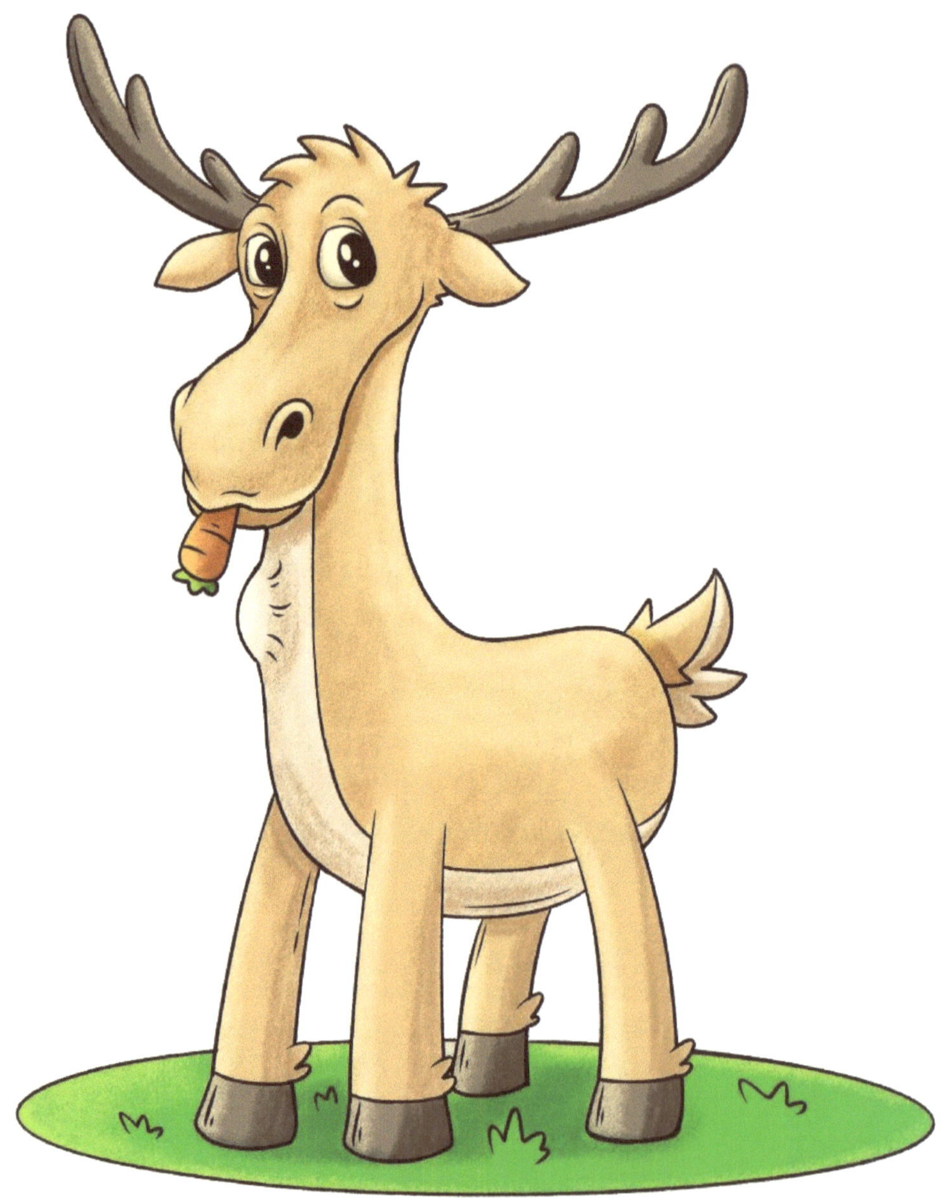

When swallowing, the lips, tongue, and cheeks should not look like
they are moving. Swallowing is done by muscles near your throat only.
The only part that you should see moving when you swallow is the
area around your Adam's Apple (on your neck).

Imagine your mouth is like a little round box
The top teeth are like the lid
The bottom teeth should neatly be stacked under it

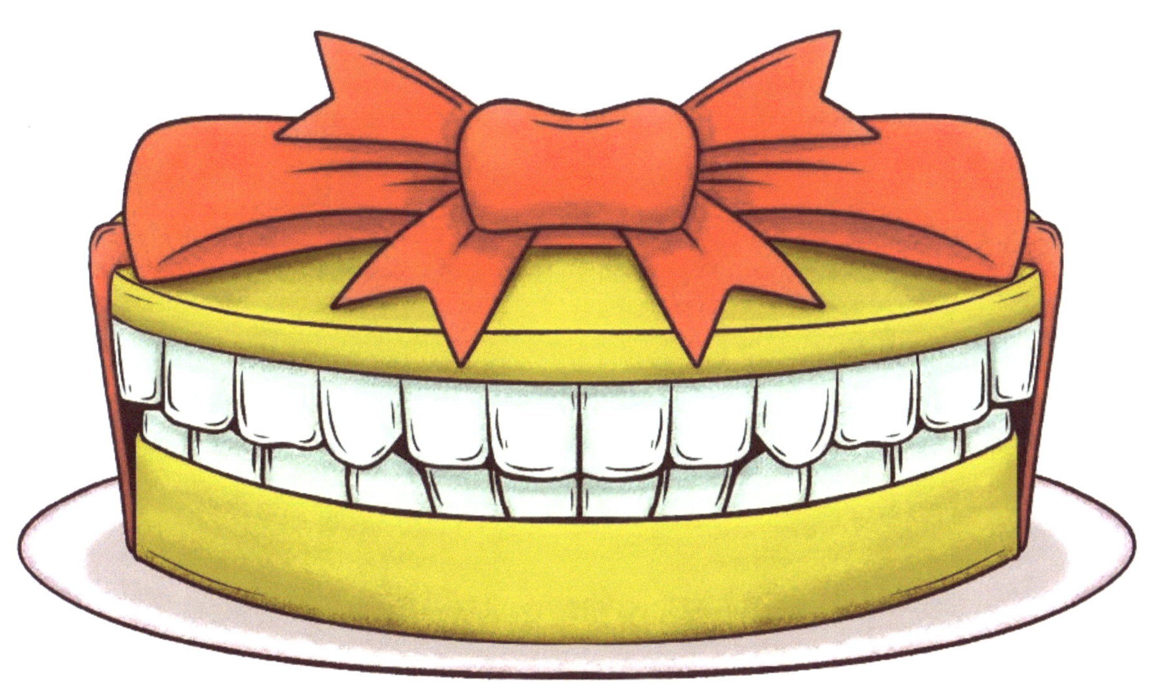

When you have healthy habits, your teeth stay straight and last for a lifetime. If the top teeth gently overlap your bottom teeth, it will protect your muscles and joints so that you will be able to enjoy eating your favourite foods all your life.

And that is how you will shape your perfect smile!

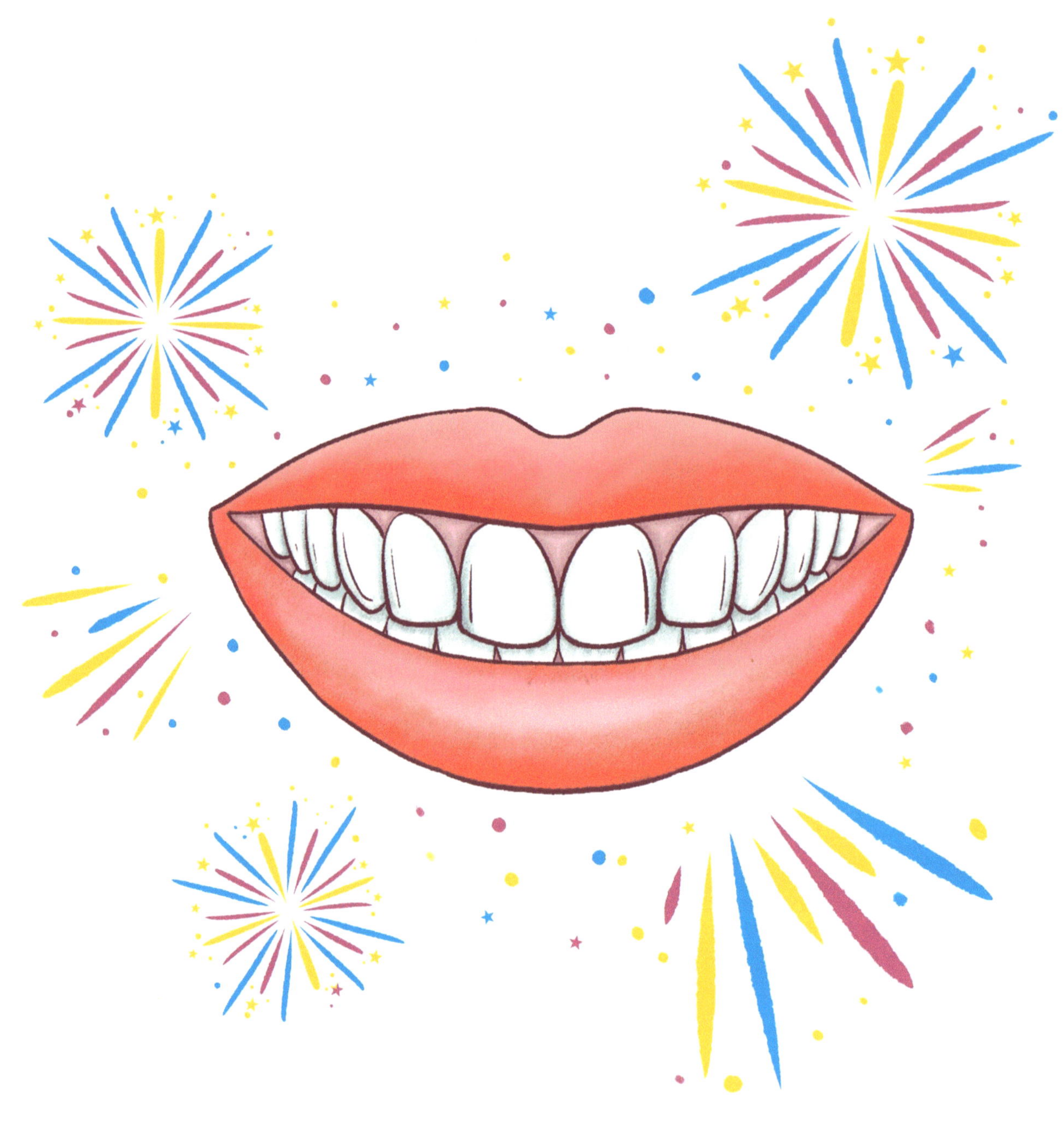

Can you remember?

1.Breathing from your <u>mouth</u> makes you
 A. Healthy
 B. Tired
 C. Hungry

2. Mouth breathing changes your <u>face</u> by
 A. Making your face look longer
 B. Make your face look wider
 C. Stay the same

3. <u>Snoring</u> means you are
 A. Tired
 B. Breathing from your mouth
 C. Breathing from your nose

4. What part of your <u>face</u> should move when you swallow?
 A. Chin
 B. Lips
 C. No part should move

5. A wrinkle on your <u>chin</u> when you chew and swallow means you are
 A. Eating fast
 B. Swallowing right
 C. Swallowing wrong

6. When you swallow, your <u>tongue</u> should
 A. Move all around
 B. Push between your teeth
 C. Stay touching the top part (roof) of your mouth

7. Sucking your lips makes your <u>teeth</u>
 A. Look nice
 B. Look like beaver teeth
 C. Change colour

8. Biting, sucking and licking <u>lips</u> will make them
 A. Beautiful
 B. Feel better
 C. Dry, red and sore

9. <u>Chewing and sucking</u> on your thumb, fingernails, or pencils will
 A. Make you feel better
 B. Make your teeth break and have gaps in them
 C. Make you less hungry

10. Grinding your <u>teeth</u> will make them
 A. Strong
 B. Break
 C. Sharp

11. Horses have straight teeth and are full of energy because they can <u>breathe</u> from
 A. Nose only
 B. Mouth only
 C. Both nose and mouth

12. Breathing from your nose makes you <u>feel</u>
 A. Tired
 B. Relaxed and happy
 C. Angry

13. When you are not using your <u>tongue</u>, it should be
 A. Sleeping in the roof of your mouth
 B. Moving all around
 C. Pushed between your lips and teeth

14. Your <u>food</u> should be
 A. Swallowed fast
 B. Chewed slowly with your back teeth
 C. Chewed hard

15. The best <u>side</u> to chew food on is
 A. Right side
 B. Left side
 C. Both left and right

16. The muscles that move when you <u>swallow</u> are
 A. Lips and tongue
 B. Cheeks
 C. Muscles at the back of your mouth only (near your throat)

Answer Key: 1-(B), 2-(A), 3-(B), 4-(C), 5-(C), 6-(C), 7(B), 8-(C), 9-(B), 10-(B), 11-(A), 12-(B), 13-(A), 14-(B), 15-(C), 16-(C)